Becoming an Activated Patient

Becoming an Activated Patient

How to Take Control and Enhance Your Level of Health Care

Alexander "Sandy" Halperin, DDS
Gina Davidson

Dedicated to
patients and health care professionals worldwide

Just when the caterpillar

thought the world was over,

it became a butterfly.

— proverb

Acknowledgments

This book represents a great deal of my life, beginning with my incredibly loving parents, Elsie and Leon. They gave me virtually everything and were the first to teach me the foundations of relationships, how to appropriately interact with others, and how to get by in the medical world during my youth.

I am most thankful for Gail, the core of my life, and for our two daughters, Karen and Lauren, our son-in-law Brett, and our three grandchildren, Emma, Rebecca and Madeline.

The effort of authoring this book would not have been possible without the support of my dear friends, doctors Steven Gallant and Lee Sheldon, my brothers, Mark and Joe, and each of their families.

A number of friends, new and old, also have been highly instrumental in helping me to deliver the messages in this book and enhancing the quality of my life: Gina and Larry Davidson, Don and Jeanette Yaeger, Margaret Farris, Bill Wertman, Pat Hogan, Everett and Marie Yarborough, Tom and Patty Betts, Lyla and Frank Ellzey, Steve Orfield, Richard Scheck, Jim and Pat Ryan, and countless others who have inspired and supported me in huge ways.

I owe far more than a big thanks to my personal health care team who are among the most talented, compassionate, intuitive, and tireless in the field:

doctors Tracey Hellgren, Angela Spencer, Ken Brummel-Smith, Akash Ghai, Bob Soni, and Rob Simpson.

Finally, without Gina, the writing of this book would never have taken place. Gina spent nearly a year interviewing me, recording my ideas, and providing a great deal of her own thoughts. Gina coming into my life during the time that I had Alzheimer's and was unable to author this book by myself has been one of the greatest gifts of my life.

— *Sandy Halperin, DDS*

◇◇◇◇◇◇◇

It has been an absolute joy to get to know the Halperin family during the writing of this book. I thank Sandy, Gail, Karen, and Lauren for welcoming me into their circle, for candidly sharing their stories, and for giving me constructive feedback as we went along. I also thank them for all the lunches, Diet Dr. Peppers, cups of coffee, and miniature Hershey bars.

Sandy and I were privileged to receive ongoing feedback and excellent editing services from members of Red Pen Writers, my local writing group. Thank you to our coach, Heather Whitaker, and to our editors Liz Jameson, Jessica Thompson, Lipika Frith, Aide Whitaker, Mary Bowers, and Tracy Sprayberry for your thoughtful advice and your considerable time. Thanks also to Dorothy Green and Maggie Beth McGrotha for reading and rereading, for endless editing, and for asking important questions that led to a better book.

A great amount of time has been needed for the research, writing, development, design, and publishing of this book, and I thank my husband Larry and our children, Ty and Jillian, for their patience and understanding during the process. A huge thank you to Larry as well for editing, helping with design, and for creating and hosting www.EnhanceYourHealthCare.com, where you can download copies of these tools.

Thank you to my parents, Sharon and Charlie Green, and to all of my wonderful family and friends who encourage me to keep writing.

And special thanks again to Sandy — for reaching out, finding me, and letting me share in this adventure.

— *Gina Davidson*

Table of Contents

Foreword

Kenneth Brummel-Smith, MD
Charlotte Edwards Maguire Professor
Department of Geriatrics Chair
Florida State University College of Medicine

You are about to embark on a remarkable journey. As I was reading Dr. Halperin's guide (we've now become friends so I'll refer to him as "Sandy"), I wrote in the margin, "This is really interesting!" He has created a practical, organized approach to managing personal health information that would certainly help any doctor caring for a patient. I am convinced that if more patients provided this type of information to their physicians, medical care would be more patient-centered, focused on individual needs, and less risky.

Medical care is undergoing significant changes. The publication of "To Err is Human" by the Institute of Medicine (IOM)[i] in 1999 shocked the world by documenting that nearly 100,000 persons die each year in the United States from preventable medical errors. In the last 10 years, there has been increasing emphasis on "patient-centered health care," which the IOM defines as "providing care that is respectful of and responsive to individual patient preferences, needs, and values, and ensuring that patient values guide all clinical decisions." [ii] Ed Wagner, MD, a member of IOM, recommended that health systems that care for people with chronic conditions do best when dealing with "an activated patient." [iii]

What better way for patients to have personal preferences and values respected and to become activated in their own course of health care than to have their preferences and values clearly documented in the comprehensive set of tools offered in this book?

Although we doctors are encouraged to use the best available scientific evidence in making medical recommendations, ultimately the right decision for an individual patient comes from the input of an informed patient combined with the wisdom and advice of the physician.

The need for accurate and up-to-date information from the patient is even more important when the patient has multiple medical conditions. In such a situation, which is now the norm for many people older than 55, the patient often sees multiple doctors and takes multiple medications. While this may be useful in many cases, it also is a recipe for potential disaster. Physicians may not communicate with one another, may be unaware of the medicines prescribed by other specialists, and may not take the time to elicit the goals and wishes of each patient. And it is often hard for a physician to get in immediate contact with another physician to clarify information. But there is one person who is always present at every medical visit — the patient!

In reality, the real primary care provider is the patient. You may see your family doctor or internist a few times a year, but if you have one or more chronic conditions, you'll be treating yourself 24/7/365. As a "back-up" primary provider, I can best assist those patients who are well informed about their own health status. With the tools Sandy has created, you will be an informed, activated patient, much more likely to have your values guide all clinical decisions. Coping and thriving with a chronic condition is sometimes a difficult journey, and any journey is much harder when you don't know where you are going. With Sandy's tools, you can chart your course and improve the quality and safety of your experience.

Maybe you think you won't be able to do this. If so, think about who authored this book. Sandy has Early Stage Alzheimer's disease. He knew that he had only a limited amount of time to get this information out to the public, and the sooner the better. In hours of talking with him, I have been struck by his indomitable desire to improve medical care for all. He is one of the most passionate advocates I have ever met. I truly believe he will do better than many with Alzheimer's because he is practicing exactly what he "preaches" in this book.

I am happy he was able to connect with Gina Davidson who assisted him in the development of this book. Her input clearly helped organize Sandy's ideas and brought out the best in his careful thinking and guidance. As you will see in the Introduction, he's even taught her a thing or two about being a more activated patient.

And I would have to say the same goes for me.

---

[i] To Err is Human, IOM Report, 1999

[ii] Crossing the Quality Chasm, IOM Report, 2001

[iii] Ed Wagner

Introduction
Gina Davidson

Sandy Halperin invited me into his life when I was two years into writing a book about my own. He was two years into living with his diagnosis of Early Stage Alzheimer's disease. In an effort to bring the idea of this health care book to fruition, he was searching for a co-author, a freelance writer, who could help him; he found me on LinkedIn, a website where professionals post their resumes and connect with other professionals.

During our first phone conversation, Sandy was candid about his history of chronic illness and told me about his cognitive impairment. I also learned he was one of 10 people in the United States chosen to be on the National Alzheimer's Association's Early Stage Advisory Group.

He shared his ideas for this book that had been on his mind for more than a decade, and for which he'd written an outline years before. But, like many of us, Sandy had other responsibilities to attend to, most importantly his family and work. And because of his chronic illnesses, his health was also a top concern. When Sandy contacted me, he was in his early '60's and at a point where he had some time to develop his ideas.

His memory was fading more quickly than he had anticipated it would, so the possibility of sharing his knowledge was becoming limited. His heart, however, faced no such obstacle.

"I know if you prompt me with questions from the outline," Sandy said during our first meeting, "I'll be able to tell you what I want people to know."

I was intrigued — partly because he had such conviction for his cause, partly because he spoke about his health setbacks with such fortitude, and partly because I knew a bit about Alzheimer's. My 90-year-old grandfather-in-law had recently succumbed to the disease. I began working at the Department of Elder Affairs shortly after his death, where I learned the clinical side of Alzheimer's and how it was affecting Floridians. And during my time there, I read *Still Alice*, a true-to-life novel from the point of view of a middle-aged woman diagnosed with Early Stage Alzheimer's.

The more I listened to Sandy's ideas, the more I believed that others needed to hear what he had to say. We journeyed into his mind and memories, culling stories from his childhood, which was filled with a love for medicine yet riddled with chronic illness. We talked about how Sandy coped through dental school and most of his adult life while battling bouts of bronchial infections. And he shared with me how Alzheimer's was changing his life. Along the way, he revealed the many health care strategies he had learned in an effort to effectively take care of himself and his family.

Over the course of many hours and months, as I inquired about each item he had listed in his outline and recorded and typed up his words, I soaked up his sincerity and passion for his purpose.

Even though I do not have a chronic or life-threatening illness, I knew that my family and I (and everyone else I knew) would benefit from hearing his words. I found I could no longer write the words without living by them. I began to write notes for my doctors. I was friendlier (and less intimidated) with the staff. I even made conversation with those in white coats, something I had never really thought to do before. I have seen terrific results from my efforts; I have greatly enhanced my own health care.

Likewise, I believe Sandy's lessons and tools can be used to improve your health care, the health care of your children, an aging parent, a chronically ill friend, or anyone.

When I first approached the Halperins' apartment back in January 2013, I couldn't help but notice the welcoming, sunny yellow lounge chairs on the balcony porch. Resting on a window ledge above the chairs was a white card with brilliant blue writing that said, "Just when the caterpillar thought the world was over, it became a butterfly." Sandy is indeed that proverbial butterfly.

Rather than being defeated by hardship and illness, Sandy's profound desire to make the world a better place prompted him to help all of us become the activated patients we need to be. His commitment to health care has led him to being an international advocate for Alzheimer's awareness and funding, and the author of this special book, which he hopes will encourage millions of people to take a greater role in their own health care.

I feel blessed to be among the first.

Preface: Finding My Way

Just after one o'clock in the morning on Thursday, February 11, 1982, my body woke me because it could no longer breathe. Startled, I sat up, my eyes immediately darting to my wife, Gail, who was asleep beside me. I opened my mouth to tell her something was wrong, but I was unable to speak. It felt as if my entire airway was blocked. I frantically gasped for air but none came.

Instinctively, I sprang to my feet and jumped up and down on our bedroom floor. When that failed to shock my body into breathing, I beat on the bedroom wall with both fists.

Breathe! I willed my body. *Breathe!*

I gasped again. No air.

With no particular plan in mind, I ran out of the room and shot down our narrow hallway toward the kitchen, knocking pictures off the walls as I went. Suddenly, I heard Gail's footsteps closing in behind me.

"Sandy!" she yelled, "What is it?"

I whipped around and grabbed at my throat in desperation.

"You can't breathe?" she shot back in response, her eyes wild with fear.

She knew my history of chronic bronchial inflammation and that I had put my health at risk earlier that week. I was a prosthodontist, specializing in dentures since determining years before that my bronchial condition worsened considerably when drilling natural teeth. Though it hadn't been medically documented, I knew that this drilling created a highly contaminated viral and bacterial aerosol that when breathed in caused the tissues in my throat to swell.

"I'm calling for help," Gail said, and ran frantically to the kitchen. She grabbed the phone receiver off the wall and dialed 911. My world began to move in slow motion as I sank to my knees and heard her give our address.

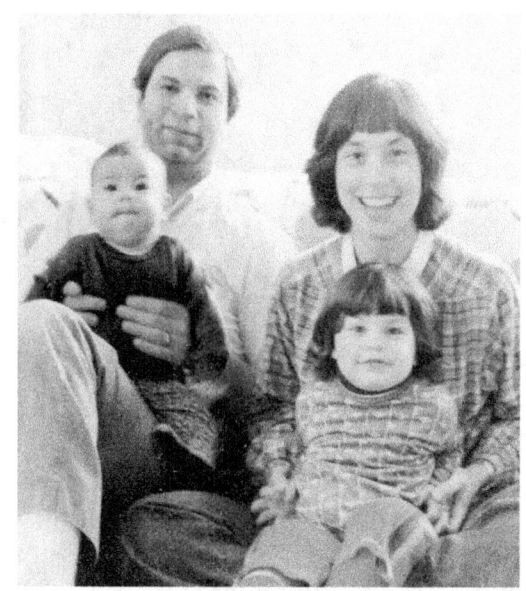

Our family, 1982

I'm going to die, I thought. *I'm not going to see my kids grow up.*

Karen was 2, and Lauren was just a baby. I could hear their cries coming from their bedrooms.

I berated myself for going against my better judgment and thought back to the patient who had needed my help earlier that week. No one else had been around to do the drilling that needed to be done.

I'd taken extra precautions — opening up windows, layering two face masks over my nose and mouth, wearing glasses to protect my eyes and Latex gloves to protect my hands. Even so, symptoms of bronchial infection had begun within half an hour, and I knew I'd made a terrible mistake.

Gail hung up the phone, glanced at me on the floor, and went to the kitchen drawer where we kept our steak knives. I looked up to find her holding one in her hand. Her eyes stared intently into mine, and I knew what she was thinking. Years before, I had read about a procedure, called a cricothyrotomy, that could be done to puncture the throat near the Adam's Apple to establish an airway. Because I had come close to losing my airway many times, I wanted to know what to do should a worst-case scenario arise. Gail let me know she'd be horrified if we ever had to do it.

She stood trembling above me with the knife in her hand, her eyes asking, "Do I have to?"

I knew from my medical training that there was only one alternative; it was possible the buildup of carbon dioxide in my blood would break the spasm in my larynx and cause my vocal chords to open. But would that happen before I stopped breathing altogether? Only a couple of minutes had passed since I'd awoken, but it felt like hours.

Sitting on my knees, drenched with sweat, I glanced up at Gail and tried to breathe again. Mercifully, miraculously, a bit of air came through. It felt like I was sucking air through a pinhole. I gasped again and again, inhaling a bit more air each time.

I had told Gail the night before that if I was ever going to die of my pulmonary problems, this might be it. How close I had come.

By the time the ambulance arrived, my airway had expanded enough for me to breathe more freely. Regardless, I was rushed to a local hospital, and then to a larger one, where I stayed for two weeks.

I spent my nights fighting sleep, afraid I would again stop breathing. To stay alert, and as I saw it "alive," I walked the silent, sterile hallways, wheeling my IV pole alongside me. After I tired of circling the nurses' station and had passed by each patient's room multiple times, I would head back to my room and mindlessly click the television remote from station to station. I talked to every nurse who came by. I knew my body would naturally wake me up again if I couldn't breathe, but I didn't want to count on it.

I still don't like to count on anything or anyone when it comes to staying alive, but I have found through the years that I have to. We all do. For our medical well-being, we have to depend on doctors, nurses, staff members, specialists, surgeons, and others. We are all in this together, but it is sometimes easy to forget that we, the patients, are as vital to the management of our health care as the professionals we visit. This is especially crucial when details about our health don't translate easily into known medical terms or diagnoses. We, the patients, carry the responsibility of communicating honestly and effectively with our doctors, and are responsible for helping to build relationships that will give us the best shot at living well.

Throughout my life, as I hopscotched from doctor to doctor, I developed tools to make office visits more productive, keep my history up to date, keep my doctors informed, and to help me be prepared in case of emergency. For many years, I have wanted to share this information in the interest of helping others. When I was diagnosed with Early Stage Alzheimer's disease, it became evident that the time to share was now.

I enlisted the help of a co-author who has interviewed me for hours on end about my struggles with illnesses, my achievements in the face of adversity, and my quest to empower others to take their health care into their own hands and communicate their needs with their team of professionals.

This book begins with me and my health, but it is ultimately for you and your health. It is my greatest hope that you will take these tools and use them to become an activated patient and a vital participant in the enhancement of your own health care. I believe the use of these tools has kept me alive and has enabled me to remain proactive and lead an active life in spite of my many medical conditions.

From my heart to yours, I offer you the opportunity to learn from my mistakes and benefit from my triumphs. Your health is literally in your hands.

Chapter 1: Taking the First Steps

In the early 1980's, a couple of years before my near-death experience, I visited a series of doctors where I was living in New York City. As I made the rounds, I developed a growing sense that I often wasn't being listened to or believed because my internal illnesses couldn't be seen. My particular bronchial condition had not yet been thoroughly studied and was not understood by the greater medical community, so I felt the need to prove myself as I told my story again and again. And I worried that the tests being done by my doctors wouldn't validate my symptoms.

I was in a world very different from the one I'd grown up in. My dad had been the owner of a neighborhood pharmacy in Springfield, Mass., and had known every physician in town, so I grew up knowing most of them by their first names. My mother and my pediatrician were close friends, and it was normal for them to sit and shoot the breeze for hours following a house call. The father of one of my childhood friends was a doctor of internal medicine and would talk with us about the intricacies of medicine, disease and treatments. So from a young age, I was fascinated with the medical professional and yearned to know more. I read every medical book I could get my hands on and immersed myself in conversations with the physicians my family knew. I learned the vernacular, gained a great deal of medical knowledge, and had access to quality care whenever I needed it.

When I left Massachusetts to go to graduate school in New York City, I didn't realize I was leaving behind medical care as I knew it. I went out into a world where physicians didn't come to my house, and would likely not even know my name if I passed them on the street.

At one point, after suffering from continual bouts of bronchial infection, I went to see a physician who was referred to me by a friend. I showed up for the appointment seriously sick, completely unprepared, and equal parts terrified and hopeful to learn the cause of my illness. I was desperate for answers and hoped the doctor would be able to give them to me.

You have the power to make the health care changes you seek. Now is the time to begin.

You can imagine my shock when the first question he asked me was, "Do you want the $50 exam, the $100 exam, or the $150 exam?"

I didn't understand his question, and I didn't know how to answer it. Was this doctor basing the thoroughness of my exam on the amount of money I could afford to pay him? What kind of question was that to ask a patient in need?

"I'm sick, and I want to get better," I finally replied, and then timidly added, "I guess I'll get the $150 exam because I don't want you to leave anything out."

Since his "thorough" exam resulted in my admittance to a nearby hospital and the battery of tests they ran led to some resolutions, I was glad I paid top dollar. I've wondered all my life if I'd still be alive if I had chosen the $50 exam.

I've come a long way since those days of feeling lost, confused, and desperate when it comes to my own health care. Because of my intense interest in the human body and my own dilapidated one, I've become an expert health care advocate by training myself to prepare for appointments, by connecting with my doctors and their staffs, and by learning how to effectively manage the emotions that come with chronic and debilitating illnesses. I've become, in effect, an activated patient.

Here's the simple truth: Your health care is not going to improve without your preparation and active participation. The time you spend before your appointment will increase the quality and efficiency of your care. Take the time you need before your medical visit to think clearly, concentrate on what you'd like to get from your appointment, and make a list for both you and your doctor to review. Thinking through what you'd like to address will increase your chances of remembering key questions and the likelihood that the conversation with your doctor will be productive. It offers you your best chance of leaving your appointment satisfied.

You have the power to make the health care changes you seek and the power to make your doctors pay attention to you.

Now is the time to begin. Get out a pen, and take a look at the first tools to get you on your way.

Tool 1: Current Symptoms

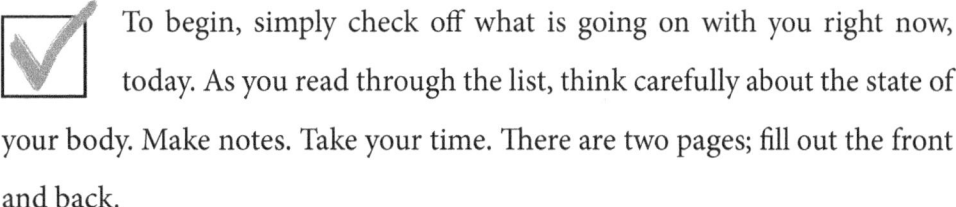 To begin, simply check off what is going on with you right now, today. As you read through the list, think carefully about the state of your body. Make notes. Take your time. There are two pages; fill out the front and back.

Tool 2: Current Medications

Time and again, we are asked for this information. Instead of racking your brain trying to remember long prescription drug names and exact doses, record them and take this with you to your visit.

A list of current medications is especially helpful should an emergency arise. Family and friends will be glad to know what you need, as will an admitting physician. And you might not be in any condition to tell them.

Tool 3: Current Physicians & Health Care Providers

It's a good idea for your doctor to know who else is on your health care team. Together, that's what they are: your team. And it might be good for you to remember their names and addresses, especially if you don't see them often. Enhancing your health care is truly as easy as 1-2-3. But you have to actually do the work to make it work.

A Note about the Tools

Tools mentioned throughout the text are located at the end of each chapter and again (in number order) at the end of the book in a section called **Tools You Can Use**. You can **make additional copies or download them at www.EnhanceYourHealthCare.com**. See that section for details.

I suggest copying tools for future use and keeping your completed tools in a binder or file for easy reference. This will make it easy for you to take them along to doctor visits and to add to your file after each visit.

You also may want to download them and keep them in a file on your computer desktop, or email a PDF to yourself for handy reference on a mobile device.

Sometimes, I simply print out my forms and submit them to the doctor's office instead of filling out their version of the same forms. Of course, always ask the office staff if the replacement forms are acceptable to your doctor.

Current Symptoms

Patient Name _____ Date _____ / _____ / _____

Head/Mental
____ Anxiety
____ Depression
____ Memory loss (long-term)
____ Memory loss (short-term)
____ Mood swings
____ Nervousness
____ Other _____

Head/Physical
____ Dizziness
____ Headaches
____ Redness in the face
____ Seizures
____ Other _____

Eyes
____ Bloody
____ Blurry vision
____ Change in vision
____ Double vision
____ Dryness
____ Floaters in eye
____ Infection
____ Itchy
____ Night blindness
____ Pain
____ Redness
____ Sensitivity to light
____ Other _____

Heart
____ Fluttering (skipping beats)
____ Pain
____ Pressure
____ Rapid heartbeat
____ Other _____

Nose
____ Bleeding
____ Dripping
____ Dryness
____ Frequent colds
____ Sneezing
____ Stuffiness
____ Other _____

Ears
____ Bleeding
____ Discharge
____ Frequent ear infections
____ Hearing problems
____ Pain
____ Redness
____ Ringing in ears
____ Waxy
____ Other _____

Mouth
____ Bad breath
____ Bleeding gums
____ Cold sores
____ Dental pain
____ Discomfort in jaw joint
____ Dryness
____ Excess saliva
____ Infection
____ Loose teeth
____ Sensitive teeth (hot/cold)
____ Sores that don't heal
____ White sores
____ Other _____

Neck
____ Neck pain/stiffness
____ Swollen lymph nodes
____ Other _____

Throat
____ Dryness
____ Difficulty swallowing
____ Difficulty speaking
____ Excessive clearing of throat
____ Frequent sore throats
____ Hoarseness
____ Mucus
____ Other _____

Chest/Breast/Lungs
____ Coughing
____ Coughing up blood
____ Coughing up mucus
____ Discolored mucus
____ Frequent colds
____ Pain or discomfort
____ Shortness of breath
____ Unusual discharge
____ Other _____

Back
____ Aches
____ Cramps
____ Pain
____ Other _____

Shoulders/Arms/Elbows/Hands
____ Numbness
____ Pain
____ Swelling
____ Tingling
____ Other _____

Allergies
_____

Current Symptoms

Patient Name _____ Date _____ / _____ / _____

Legs/Knees

____ Cramps
____ Pain
____ Swelling
____ Tingling
____ Other _____

Ankles/Feet

____ Burning
____ Dryness
____ Flaking
____ Itchy
____ Numbness
____ Pain
____ Sores that won't heal
____ Swelling
____ Toe pain
____ Other _____

Skin

____ Dryness
____ Hives
____ Itchy
____ Moles that changed color
____ Rashes
____ Sores
____ Sores that don't heal

Urinary Tract

____ Blood in urine
____ Burning/painful urination
____ Difficulty urinating
____ Frequent urinary infections
____ Frequent urination
____ Incontinence
____ Other

Nails

____ Brittle
____ Change in color
____ Fungus
____ Other _____

Gastrointestinal

____ Abdominal pain
____ Blood in stool
____ Change in bowels
____ Constipation
____ Diarrhea
____ Heartburn
____ Hemorrhoids
____ Nausea
____ Poor appetite
____ Reflux
____ Tarry stool
____ Vomiting
____ Vomiting up blood
____ Other _____

Reproductive System

____ Bleeding
____ Change in flow
____ Irregular menstrual cycle
____ No periods
____ Pain
____ Staining
____ Testicular pain
____ Unusual discharge
____ Other _____

General

____ Anemia
____ Difficulty balancing
____ Dizziness
____ Easy bruising or bleeding
____ Excessive sweating

____ Excessive thirst
____ Fainting
____ Fatigue
____ Fevers/chills
____ Frequent urination
____ Heat or cold intolerance
____ Hot flashes
____ Involuntary movements
____ Joint pain
____ Lightheaded
____ Limited range of motion
____ Muscular pain
____ Need to sleep upright
____ Numbness
____ Pain
____ Recent weight gain
____ Recent weight loss
____ Shortness of breath/rest
____ Shortness of breath/exertion
____ Swollen glands
____ Trauma to a specific area
____ Tremors
____ Trouble sleeping
____ Weakness
____ Other _____

On a scale of 1-10 (1 is lowest, 10 is highest), rate your current level of pain for each symptom.

_____

_____

_____

_____

Current Medications

Patient Name _____   Date _____ / _____ / _____

Medication Name Rx #	Dosage Times/Day	When Taken	Prescribing Doctor	Reason for Taking	Notes/Side Effects/Allergies

Current Medications, Tool 2

Current Physicians & Health Care Providers

Patient Name _____ Date _____ / _____ / _____

Doctor's Name: _____ Specialty: _____

Address: _____ Phone Number: _____

Doctor's Name: _____ Specialty: _____

Address: _____ Phone Number: _____

Doctor's Name: _____ Specialty: _____

Address: _____ Phone Number: _____

Doctor's Name: _____ Specialty: _____

Address: _____ Phone Number: _____

Doctor's Name: _____ Specialty: _____

Address: _____ Phone Number: _____

Doctor's Name: _____ Specialty: _____

Address: _____ Phone Number: _____

Doctor's Name: _____ Specialty: _____

Address: _____ Phone Number: _____

Doctor's Name: _____ Specialty: _____

Address: _____ Phone Number: _____

Chapter 2: Staying Out of the Ditch

"What is the most dangerous place in the universe?"

This was one of the best questions ever asked of me in a medical setting. I'd been talking to a psychologist about managing my pain when he brought up this seemingly out-of-place question.

"What?" I asked. *What did the most dangerous place in the universe have to do with the way I was feeling?*

"Well?" He looked deeply into my eyes and waited for my response.

"The place between your ears!" he finally said. "Your brain! It's the most dangerous place in the universe!"

Oh, I thought. I began to see where he was headed.

"Why, your brain will run you into a ditch if you let it," he continued. "It'll steer you into the worst possible place every time, because that's its default setting."

Something inside of me clicked, and I knew he was right. I knew I had to stop driving myself mentally into the ditch; stop thinking about the worst possible scenarios; stop dwelling on negativity. I needed to steer my thoughts in a more positive direction. *But how*, I wondered.

He smiled as if he had read my mind.

"Drop the ugly," he said and looked intently into my eyes once more. "We go where we focus."

I left his office with new resolve and wrote down everything he said in a journal that I referred to many times over the years when worries about my illnesses would veer me mentally off course. His words of wisdom gave me strength and hope.

Drop the ugly and stay out of the ditch.

So, let's take stock of your current emotions. Are you relaxed? Feeling good? Chances are if you're suffering from an acute or chronic ailment, or fear a troublesome diagnosis, you won't be in the best of spirits — and your mind and body know it.

You're bound to have some level of anxiety or anticipation before each doctor visit, possibly the night before, and maybe even throughout the days leading up to those visits.

Feel more in control, more relaxed, and better prepared to discuss your top concerns.

As if that pressure isn't enough, when you enter the doctor's office, you're often asked to fill out forms that you may or may not know the best answers to. After waiting in the lobby, sometimes long enough to read every magazine AND catch up on Facebook, you'll typically find yourself seated in a sterile, chilly room flooded with fluorescent lighting wearing a flimsy cotton gown that never seems to cover your body completely. Underneath, you are naked, or nearly so, adding a feeling of complete vulnerability to your list of current conditions.

All of these things can lead to an increase of tension, stress, and fear. Your doctor might see this as the root of your medical condition rather than relating it to the anxiety caused by the appointment itself. If you believe you are suffering from something more than anxiety, it's important your condition is documented and brought to your doctor's attention clearly, concisely, and in writing.

Being armed with the tools in this book will help you feel more in control, more relaxed, and better prepared to discuss your top concerns. In short, it will make you feel empowered. Not only will you communicate more easily with your doctors, you'll heighten the level of your communication. And you'll get results that honestly may change your life.

Once your doctor sees you as a proactive patient, he/she may be more attentive, which will make subsequent visits more productive and less frustrating than they otherwise might be — for both you and your physician.

Both of you want you to feel better. Really.

Tool 4: My Personal Top 10 List

In addition to using the tools to help you feel more confident and in control, it's important to enjoy the time you have outside of the medical arena. You can move a step in that direction by taking a few minutes to fill out **Tool 4: My Personal Top 10 List**. Your answers — and thoughts as you decide on your answers — will serve as inspiration to focus on the many things you love to do but don't take the time to do.

In order to relieve some of your pain, stress, and fear, it's helpful to think positive thoughts and focus on pleasurable things. You can't be expected to feel happy all the time, but you can give yourself permission to take a break and do things to comfort yourself. Choosing not to dwell on the negative can ease your anxiety as you prepare for your appointment, and will help take the pressure off of you during the visit.

My psychologist encouraged me to live for what was good in the present moment, and he helped me figure out how: by keeping my brain busy doing the things I most enjoy.

Go ahead. Get busy!

My Personal Top 10 List

Name _____ Date _____ / _____ / _____

Three things I love to do but haven't done in more than a year

1. _____

2. _____

3. _____

Pick one and do it this month.

If I were invisible for a day, where would I go and what would I do?

4. _____

Consider going there and doing that.

Three friends I would love to spend the day with

5. _____

6. _____

7. _____

Call or write them and choose one day to spend with each, or get them all together.

Three things I loved to do as a kid

8. _____

9. _____

10. _____

Do them now.

Chapter 3: Prepping for Visits

In 2010, my primary care physician in Florida referred me to a neurologist to diagnose my short- and long-term memory problems. I'd been having trouble recalling information at work. Part of my job as a dental consultant included reading and commenting on patient records, and subsequently reviewing my findings with colleagues. Over and over again, within moments after closing a file, I found I couldn't remember what I'd just read. Before each meeting, I would quickly scan back through the paperwork, hoping key words would spark my memory, and I would be able to intelligently contribute to the conversation. When this no longer worked, I knew it was time to get help.

I knew I was having trouble in other areas as well. I would forget magazine stories I'd read right after reading them. I'd forget the names of people I knew well. And I would completely lose my train of thought if someone interrupted me while I was speaking. All of it was disturbing to say the least.

I went to see the neurologist my doctor recommended, and then two more just for good measure. At each of the three appointments — where I had high hopes that someone would be able to tell me what was happening to me — I showed up and winged it. Let me be clear. By winging it, I mean I showed up with no notes, no list of the medications I was taking, no list of symptoms

I was experiencing. I knew better, but I didn't follow through.

"Doctor, I have a short-term memory problem," I offered, and in my head, I finished the thought: *Please fix it.*

There were numerous questions to be answered and each appointment dragged on as I struggled to remember the details each doctor asked for.

"What medications are you taking?"

"Um, good question." I'd reply. "Let me think...."

While occasionally forgetting details doesn't mean you have a cognitive memory problem, it's still a good idea to write things down. In my case, it was even more imperative. Yet, I didn't do it. It was another thing on my to-do list, made all the more difficult because I was going to the appointments to find out why it was so difficult to do this type of thing in the first place.

Because I didn't prepare for those meetings, and because of my short-term memory problems, I was at a total loss. With no notes to guide me, I found it difficult to explain what I was going through or what I was forgetting on a daily basis. Swirling in my head was a long list of things I knew I was no longer able to do, but verbalizing them to the doctors was nearly impossible.

I left all three appointments saying to myself, *"You didn't tell them all you could have told them. How are they going to help you if you don't tell them what's wrong?"* These were three neurologists, at three separate appointments, and I didn't prepare for any of them.

Going on the scant bit of information I did provide, they each ordered neuropsychological tests to determine the extent of my cognitive capabilities. Because I hadn't written down my symptoms, the doctors needed to judge my condition based on the tests alone, and then use them to come up with what they thought was the most correct diagnosis.

Two years later, when I was asked by the local Alzheimer's Association to speak about my symptoms of Early Stage Alzheimer's, I knew I wouldn't be able to wing it. Even though for many years of my life I gave hour-long lectures without any notes, I knew there was no way I would remember what to say. This forced me to get my act together.

Over the course of a few days, I typed up a list of 25 things I was no longer able to do because of my condition. When I finished, I couldn't help but stare at the list in amazement, not because it had been such a challenge to complete but because I realized that if I had made the effort to write the list two years earlier, before my visits with the neurologists, I could have given them so much more relevant information. I could clearly see the significance of being prepared for each future appointment, whether it was a visit with a doctor or a speaking engagement.

As a patient, it's vital to remember that our doctors are relying on us for information — just like we are relying on them for answers. They practice the art of medicine, and we have to practice the art of being an active patient. What we experience on a daily basis with our medical condition is often as important as the results of any diagnostic tests a doctor might order. It's re-al-life information that can help diagnose the problem, and may lead to finding a solution or treatments more quickly.

It's vital to remember that our doctors are relying on us for information — just like we are relying on them for answers.

When you don't gather your thoughts before an appointment, you'll likely find that the visit will take longer and be less effective. If you're not prepared to answer questions, there's increased pressure as you struggle to remember everything you want to say and your providers may not get all the information they need. This makes it trickier for them to give you a proper diagnosis. Poor planning on your part will no doubt lead to more questions on your doctor's part and perhaps create a less relaxed atmosphere while you try to squeeze in all of your concerns in the limited time of your visit.

Throwing your scattered thoughts together does not often — if ever — lead to clear, concise communication in any setting. Instead, it typically leads to frustration and disappointment, especially after it's too late and you find that your poor communication has had unsatisfactory results. When it comes to doctor visits, this can lead to feelings of anger and depression.

Instead of showing up empty-handed and hoping the doctor will figure out what's wrong with you, take a few minutes to look over **Tool 1: Current Symptoms** and then think about what is most important for you to share with your doctor.

Tool 5: Health Care Visit

List these top concerns on **Tool 5: Health Care Visit**. This simple tool is one of the top ways you can get the most out of your appointment. Make a copy of **Tool 5: Health Care Visit** for your doctor and keep a copy for yourself. Bring both copies to your appointment. Give one to the receptionist, or the nurse, or directly to your doctor. It's your ticket to being listened to. It's an easy way for both of you to keep track of your top concerns and the ideal place for you to jot down notes on the suggestions and explanations your doctor gives you.

It will also make you a better listener, as you intently comprehend what's being said. And it will help you follow your doctor's orders, since you have a much better chance of remembering them.

Tool 6: Typical Daily Symptoms

In order to share your medical condition, it's beneficial to know what impact your illness/ailment/injury is having on your life. Your doctor needs to know, and so do you. On **Tool 6: Typical Daily Symptoms**, simply record what happens on a typical day, hour by hour, including before and after meals and during the night. Look for patterns (i.e., an upset stomach after breakfast each morning) and/or clues of cause-and-effect (i.e., taking medication on an empty stomach leads to nausea).

Do certain activities bring on pain? Are you taking supplements or vitamins or antibiotics? Do you drink alcohol? Caffeine? Do you smoke? Do you eat dairy? What's your sleep schedule like? How about your exercise routine?

By bringing your daily struggles into your doctor's focus, a pattern or thought might emerge, and you may hit on something you hadn't thought of before. It's all about giving relevant information.

It's your life. It's your health. Share it with the people who might be able to make it better.

Health Care Visit

Patient Name _____ Appt. Date ___ / ___ / ___

Name of Health Care Provider _____ Appt. Time _____

Address _____ Phone _____

Top Concerns
1.
Notes/Recommendations:
2.
Notes/Recommendations:
3.
Notes/Recommendations:
4.
Notes/Recommendations:
5.
Notes/Recommendations:
Conclusions/Follow-up needed:

Health Care Visit

Name _____ Doctor's Name _____ Date ____ / ____ / ____

Diet _____

_____

_____

Exercise _____

_____

_____

Lifestyle modifications (Sleep, stress reduction, etc.) _____

_____

_____

Medications (What to take, dosage, when and how long to take it, side effects, managing side effects)

_____

_____

Call doctor if _____

_____

_____

When to schedule next appointment _____

Referrals _____

_____

Additional notes _____

_____

_____

_____

Typical Daily Symptoms

Name _____ Date _____ / _____ / _____

Time	Symptoms	Notes
5-6 a.m.		
6-7 a.m.		
7-8 a.m.		
8-9 a.m.		
9-10 a.m.		
10-11 a.m.		
11 a-12 p		
12-1 p.m.		
1-2 p.m.		
2-3 p.m.		
3-4 p.m.		
4-5 p.m.		
5-6 p.m.		
6-7 p.m.		
7-8 p.m.		
8-9 p.m.		
9-10 p.m.		
10-11 p.m.		
11-12 p.m.		
12 p -3 a		
3-4 a.m.		
4-5 a.m.		

Chapter 4: Connecting with the Staff

"I can't get the specialist's clinic to call me back," I told Gail, after my third attempt to make an appointment at a doctor's office in town. This followed an initial attempt by my primary care physician, who had made an emergency referral and even placed a call herself to try to get me scheduled immediately. I had had another serious bronchial infection and was fed up with waiting for the specialist to get back with me.

"That's the place where I had trouble getting an appointment," Gail said, reminding me of the countless calls she had made with no success. I remembered her leaving messages and being upset every day the clinic didn't respond.

"We'll get back to you", they told her on the days she was fortunate enough to talk to a human being on the other end. And so she waited like I was waiting, continuing to suffer and staring at the phone.

"How'd you finally get in?" I asked, knowing that eventually she did.

Her answer was so simple; I wondered why I hadn't thought of it.

"I went there," she said, "I walked in and talked to one of the receptionists, and she gave me an appointment for that week."

There is something to be said for making personal contact, especially today when so much business is handled via mobile phones and the Internet. There is great value in making personal connections with your doctor's staff.

When you make a doctor appointment, the staff members are the first people you communicate with. They're the ones who assist you, arrange your appointments, help manage your insurance and billing, and communicate with you between visits. They can squeeze you in or not. The staff is your most important link to your doctor and an integral part of your medical team. Improving communication with your doctor begins with them.

While a phone call is quick and easy, and typically works, it may not always be the most efficient or effective method to schedule an appointment or to handle certain issues. When the situation calls for it, consider stopping by the office. This may not be as convenient, but going in person might give you an advantage because you'll have the opportunity to meet some of the staff, and this might possibly result in securing an appointment or getting you in earlier than previously scheduled. Do be mindful that the doctor is running a busy office, so be respectful of the staff's time. After all, you are one of many people who need the doctor's services.

The staff is the most important link to your doctor and an integral part of your medical team.

On the day of your appointment, do the staff (and yourself) a favor by arriving early. You'll be more relaxed, available to fill out any additional paperwork, and you might even get in ahead of time. Bring your insurance card, know your Social Security Number, and be prepared to pay.

Tool 7: Personal Health History
Tool 8: Family Health History

To further help yourself out, come with documentation of your health history, including a history of any health conditions your family members have or have had. At nearly every visit, you're asked to list this potentially critical information that could lead to a more proper diagnosis.

Take time now to record it. The information is formatted in various ways; use whichever works best for you, or use them all.

In addition to getting the facts right (you can check with other family members for accuracy if needed), you'll be able to whiz through any office paperwork. If you can get the papers in advance of your appointment, do so. Many offices will send the papers ahead of time or will let you know where to find them on their website. Take advantage of these opportunities. If they don't mention them, ask. The staff will appreciate how prepared you are, and being prepared will help you feel more in control and confident at your visit.

Your childhood health history and your family's health history may hold some surprises — better to know them now. You may also be surprised by how much you remember and how much your body has been through. This compilation of your health history is important to your doctors in determining current conditions and warding off potential problems. Be accurate and thorough, and keep it up to date.

Should an emergency arise, your loved ones will appreciate the work you've done. Better yet, share it with them ahead of time.

Personal Health History

Patient Name _____   Date _____ / _____ / _____

Previous and Current Conditions
Year condition began (and ended, if applicable)

_____ Allergies	_____ Hearing loss	_____ Obesity
_____ Alzheimer's disease	_____ Heartburn	_____ Osteopenia
_____ Anemia	_____ Heart disease	_____ Osteoporosis
_____ Arthritis	_____ Hernia	_____ Pacemaker
_____ Anxiety	_____ High blood pressure	_____ Parkinson's disease
_____ Asthma	_____ HIV	_____ Pelvic pain
_____ Back pain	_____ Incontinence	_____ Pregnancy difficulties
_____ Blood disease	_____ Infection	_____ Respiratory problems
_____ Cancer	_____ Staph infection	_____ Sciatica
_____ Cataract	_____ Infertility problems	_____ Seizures
_____ Chemical dependency	_____ Joint problems	_____ Shingles
_____ Circulation problems	_____ Joint replacement	_____ Sleep difficulties
_____ Constipation	_____ Kidney problems	_____ Swelling
_____ Depression	_____ Liver problems	_____ Thyroid problems
_____ Diabetes	_____ Memory loss (long-term)	_____ Tooth sensitivity
_____ Emphysema	_____ Memory loss (short-term)	_____ Tuberculosis
_____ Emotional disorders	_____ Mental illness	_____ Vision problems
_____ Fractures	_____ Migraines	_____ Weakness
_____ Genital disease	_____ Miscarriage	_____ Weight gain (significant)
_____ Glaucoma	_____ Multiple sclerosis	_____ Weight loss (significant)
_____ Headaches	_____ Numbness	_____ Other _____

Injury History

Injury _____   Year _____   Injury _____   Year _____

Injury _____   Year _____   Injury _____   Year _____

Injury _____   Year _____   Injury _____   Year _____

Surgery History

Surgery _____   Year _____   Surgery _____   Year _____

Surgery _____   Year _____   Surgery _____   Year _____

Surgery _____   Year _____   Surgery _____   Year _____

Personal Health History

Patient Name _____ Date _____ / _____ / _____

Chronological list of allergies, conditions, injuries, surgeries, etc.	**Age**	**Approximate date**
Begin with the most recent	_____	_____
_____	_____	_____
_____	_____	_____
_____	_____	_____
_____	_____	_____
_____	_____	_____
_____	_____	_____
_____	_____	_____
_____	_____	_____
_____	_____	_____
_____	_____	_____
_____	_____	_____
_____	_____	_____
_____	_____	_____
_____	_____	_____
_____	_____	_____
_____	_____	_____
_____	_____	_____
_____	_____	_____
_____	_____	_____

Family Health History

Patient Name _____ Date _____ / _____ / _____

_____ Anemia	_____ Glaucoma	_____ Obesity
_____ Allergies	_____ Headaches	_____ Osteopenia
_____ Alzheimer's disease	_____ Hearing loss	_____ Osteoporosis
_____ Arthritis	_____ Heart condition	_____ Pacemaker
_____ Asthma	_____ Heart disease	_____ Parkinson's disease
_____ Anxiety	_____ High blood pressure	_____ Pregnancy difficulties
_____ Back Pain	_____ HIV	_____ Respiratory problems
_____ Blood Disease	_____ Staph infections	_____ Sciatica
_____ Cancer	_____ Joint problems	_____ Seizures
_____ Cataract	_____ Joint replacement	_____ Shingles
_____ Chemical dependency	_____ Kidney problems	_____ Sleep Difficulties
_____ Circulation problems	_____ Liver problems	_____ Thyroid problems
_____ Depression	_____ Memory loss (long-term)	_____ Tuberculosis
_____ Diabetes	_____ Memory loss (short-term)	_____ Vision problems
_____ Emotional disorders	_____ Mental illness	_____ Weight gain (significant)
_____ Emphysema	_____ Miscarriage	_____ Weight Loss (significant)
_____ Genital disease	_____ Multiple sclerosis	_____ Other _____

Notes _____

_____

_____

_____

_____

On the back, write your family health history according to the family members affected.
Having this list in both forms gives you easy references depending on the way you're asked for the information.

Family Member	Full Name	Age	Health Status	Cause of death/age, if applicable
Mother				
Maternal grandmother				
Maternal grandfather				
Aunts, uncles, cousins with notable conditions				
Father				
Paternal grandmother				
Paternal grandfather				
Aunts, uncles, cousins with notable conditions				
My siblings				

Chapter 5: Communicating with Your Doctor

In 2009, before my thoughts were centered on my short- and long-term memory loss, I was suffering from multiple other medical conditions and made an appointment at a major medical center for a thorough diagnosis and recommendation of treatments. At my initial visit, I presented a primary care physician with a copy of what I call my "Body Chart." On a single page, I had comprehensively compiled all of my symptoms and conditions, giving that doctor immediate answers to many of the questions he would have asked me, saving us both time and energy.

"Can I have a copy of this?" he asked me, not only because he wanted it for my records but because of the value he saw in the chart itself. In all of his years of practice, he said, he had never had a patient present their health history that way.

Because I had efficiently detailed my symptoms and previous diagnoses on my Body Chart, there was no need for a generic question-and-answer session, which allowed us to spend the bulk of our time together digging deeper into my conditions and concerns. My doctor was able to focus on my immediate needs and quickly determine which tests and specialists would be of greatest benefit to me. He ordered the diagnostic exams and wrote the referrals for specialists I could see that week at the clinic. The next morning, I reported at 6:30 a.m. to have 25 vials of my blood taken for the testing, and soon after, began meeting with the specialists I had hoped to see.

Being prepared for the meeting with the primary doctor enabled me to relay my most pressing concerns in an organized, articulate manner, which helped me receive the excellent quality of care I was seeking. Because of my preparation and my doctor's willingness to listen, my week at the clinic was hugely productive.

Since that time, I've presented my Body Chart to numerous doctors who have been equally intrigued by it and have passed it on to other health care professionals. Nearly all of my doctors have told me how much they appreciate my preparation and how nice it would be if every patient showed up with a chart like mine.

Tool 9: Current Symptoms Body Chart

Use this tool to create your own Body Chart. The way you prepare for your appointments can make a huge difference in the quality of care you receive. Instead of arriving empty-handed, think about how much better you would feel armed with information your doctor can readily use: this chart, your current symptoms, your health history, and your list of medications and doctors.

Use Tool 1: Current Symptoms as a reference, and transfer your current symptoms to **Tool 9: Current Symptoms Body Chart** to create a comprehensive, visual tool you can share with your doctor. I've included mine at the end of this book as an example.

All of these tools serve the purpose of opening lines of communication and strengthening your relationship with your doctor. Combined, they are the life of your body, and done with care they can truly help you on your path to enhanced health care.

In addition to your list of current symptoms and concerns, you might want to give your Body Chart to the receptionist when you first arrive, or to your nurse or medical assistant when you reach the examination room. Giving it to one of them will allow your doctor to possibly review it before seeing you. If you're asked to keep it with you, that's fine too. Regardless of when you share it, the important thing is that you're prepared to talk about your specific symptoms and why you are there.

When you and your doctor each have a copy to look at, it's easy to keep your priorities in order and keep your discussion on track. It's helpful for each of you to have a visual image of what you are referring to. Many people are visual learners. The forms you share are golden communication tools that provide clarity and focus.

The forms you share are golden communication tools that provide clarity and focus.

Another way to enhance your relationship is to remember to treat your doctor like any other person. Wearing a white jacket doesn't make somebody a "god." Doctors have feelings. They get sick. They work and play every day just like you and me, and they have the same cares and concerns.

A simple "Hello," "Good to see you today," or "It's a pleasure to meet you," can go a long way. If it's your first visit, share how you found out about the office. "I was referred to you by (a family member, friend or another physician)." Or express your appreciation. "I've been looking forward to meeting with you today because...."

In doing these things, you're establishing a mutually beneficial line of communication with your doctor, which only makes sense given that you're entrusting this person with your health, your body, your life — even if it's only for one visit. You have likely established relationships with others you receive services from: your hairdresser, barber, auto mechanic, or babysitter, just to name a few. This is no different.

Another relationship builder is simple courtesy. Let the doctor know up front, "Whatever extra time you can give me will be most appreciated." If you know ahead of time that your concerns may take a while to address, let the staff know so they can adjust the doctor's schedule or let you know if it's not possible that particular day. Doctors have only a limited amount of time with each patient; be respectful when asking for special requests.

To make the staff or your doctor aware of the time you spent preparing for your appointment, let them know when you hand over your charts. Say, "I took some time to prepare for today's visit, and I want to share these with you." How can they not pay attention to that?

During your visit, use your copies as a guide, and be sure to bring along a pen to write down what the doctor says about your symptoms, concerns, and treatment options. Don't expect to remember everything that's said.

Ask questions until they've all been answered, and the answers are clear to you. Make sure you understand any instructions, so you can be compliant with your doctor's orders.

You'll likely want to share this information later with family or friends. Better yet, bring someone with you. It's great to have another set of ears in the room, and may make it possible for you to take better notes and focus on what your doctor is saying.

If your doctor refers you to another doctor or specialist, you may want to ask, "Where would you go to get this taken care of? Where would you send your spouse?" It's worth a try.

Be sure to research any referral, including asking friends and family who they prefer and why. You may want to have an idea of which doctor you would prefer to see before the staff asks you (provided there's a choice in your community). If you know ahead of time that your symptoms may warrant a referral, find out who is available to you, and go to your appointment knowing your preference. Waiting to get an appointment with a doctor you know you'd like to go to is far wiser than starting with one you don't know or may find out you don't want. Trying to switch down the road might be complicated.

As your visit winds down, pause for a moment to be sure you said everything you wanted to say and that you feel satisfied. That way, you won't later dwell on things you didn't say, you won't need to call the office back, and you won't need to set up a subsequent visit to finish your thoughts.

Before your doctor leaves the room, ask, "Am I going to see you again today?" Sometimes the visit is over before you know it.

Ask if your charts can be added to your medical record, and be sure to express your appreciation. It's as simple as saying, "Thank you for your time."

Before you leave the office, check in with the staff to make a follow-up appointment if necessary. This will save you from having to call back to schedule an appointment later. Also, periodically ask for a copy of any pertinent records you may want to keep in your personal files or a health care binder (CT scans, x-rays, MRIs, blood tests, etc., including diagnostic reports).

Periodically ask for a copy of any pertinent records you may want to keep in your personal files.

After your visit, take a few minutes to reflect on it. See **Tool 5: Health Care Visit**. Take time to jot down notes while you're in the waiting area or in your car, when you have the best chance of remembering the details. Make a note of your doctor's responses to your top concerns and think about the recommendations that were offered.

Tool 10: Evaluation Form

Take a closer look at the care you receive. You have every right to evaluate your doctor and the staff. On the back, rate yourself as a patient. It may help you focus on things you can improve on at future visits.

Finally, if you are prescribed a new medication or you visit with a new doctor, be sure to update **Tool 2: Current Medications** and **Tool 3: Current Physicians & Health Care Providers**.

Current Symptoms

Patient Name _____ Date _____

My Front Left Side

My Front Right Side

_____

_____

_____

_____

_____

_____

_____

_____

_____

_____

_____

_____

_____

_____

_____

_____

Current Symptoms Body Chart, Tool 9 — 1 of 2

Current Symptoms

Patient Name _____ Date _____

My Back Left Side

_____
_____
_____
_____
_____
_____
_____
_____
_____
_____
_____
_____
_____
_____
_____
_____
_____
_____

My Back Right Side

_____
_____
_____
_____
_____
_____
_____
_____
_____
_____
_____
_____
_____
_____
_____
_____
_____

Evaluation Form (Office Visit)

Doctor's Name _____ Appt. Date ____ / ____ / ____

Address _____ Specialty _____

Rating the Office Visit				
Reception				
1. How many minutes I waited to be seen	0-15 mins.	15-30 mins.	30-45 mins.	45+ mins.
2. How many minutes I waited once in the room	0-15 mins.	15-30 mins.	30-45 mins.	45+ mins.
1= Disagree, 2 = Somewhat agree, 3 = Agree, 4 = Strongly agree				
3. I was warmly greeted by the staff.	1	2	3	4
4. I was warmly greeted by the doctor.	1	2	3	4
5. The doctor respectfully accepted my prepared forms.	1	2	3	4
6. The doctor paid attention to my medical issue(s).	1	2	3	4
7. The doctor addressed my top concerns.	1	2	3	4
8. The doctor validated my medical concerns.	1	2	3	4
Communication Skills				
1= Inadequate, 2= Adequate, 3 = Better than average, 4 = Excellent				
1. Listened attentively	1	2	3	4
2. Seemed caring and compassionate	1	2	3	4
3. Exhibited acceptable "bedside manner"	1	2	3	4
4. Answered all my questions appropriately	1	2	3	4
5. Interacted well with office staff	1	2	3	4
6. Treated my family/friends well	1	2	3	4
Clinical Skills				
1= Inadequate, 2= Adequate, 3 = Better than average, 4 = Excellent				
1. Spent an adequate amount of time with me	1	2	3	4
2. Quality of the clinical examination	1	2	3	4
3. Management of my medical issues	1	2	3	4
4. Diagnostic skills and clinical judgment	1	2	3	4
5. Made appropriate referrals, if needed	1	2	3	4
Will you see this doctor again? Yes No (If no, keep this for records in case you are referred in the future.)				
If not, why not?				
Comments regarding office staff:				
Additional comments:				

Evaluation Form (Myself)

Doctor's Name _____ Appt. Date ____ / ____ / ____

Address _____ Specialty _____

Rating Myself		
Preparation		
1. Time of appointment:		
2. Time I arrived:		
3. Completed paperwork prior to visit, if requested	Yes	No
4. Arrived early to fill out paperwork, if needed	Yes	No
5. Complied with all preparation requests prior to visit	Yes	No
6. Brought completed Tool 1: Current Symptoms	Yes	No
7. Brought completed Tool 2: Current Medications	Yes	No
8. Brought completed Tool 3: Current Physicians & Health Care Providers	Yes	No
9. Brought completed Tool 5: Health Care Visit	Yes	No
10. Brought completed Tool 6: Typical Daily Symptoms	Yes	No
11. Brought completed Tool 7: Personal Health History	Yes	No
12. Brought completed Tool 8: Family Health History	Yes	No
13. Brought completed Tool 9: Current Symptoms Body Chart	Yes	No
14. Brought completed Tool 12: Checklist for Tests, Procedures & Surgeries, if needed	Yes	No
15. Brought completed Tool 13: Daily Medications, if needed	Yes	No
At the Visit		
1. Communicated effectively with the staff	Yes	No
2. Gave doctor/staff a copy of my tool(s)	Yes	No
3. Voiced each concern	Yes	No
4. Completed front Tool 5: Health Care Visit	Yes	No
5. Made follow-up appointment, if needed	Yes	No
After the Visit		
1. Completed Tool 10: Evaluation of Office Visit	Yes	No
2. Completed back of Tool 5: Health Care Visit	Yes	No
3. Completed Tool 11: Post-Visit Action Plan	Yes	No
What I could have done differently to make the appointment more productive:		

Chapter 6: Following Your Doctor's Orders

During my career as a clinical and academic dentist, I was involved in the treatment of thousands of patients, including some who did not tell me the truth about the frequency of their brushing and flossing. It was apparent to me, however, that many of them had not been cleaning on a routine basis and had vigilantly brushed their teeth just prior to their appointment with me.

Even though my oral examination revealed they had not been practicing proper oral hygiene, I would casually ask them, "How much time do you spend each day brushing and flossing your teeth?"

Many patients thought their last-minute brushing would hide their poor habits from me, and many would give me a generally acceptable answer. But when probed with a few more questions — as I was probing their bleeding gums — most would sheepishly own up to the fact that they had not been completely compliant.

Since I was keenly aware of the truth anyway, I was appreciative when patients let me know they weren't following the instructions I'd recommended. Their open, honest communication with me was refreshing and enabled me to know how to best continue their treatment.

Your doctors want the same from you. If you're not following their instructions, just tell them. Don't try to fake it. Chances are your doctors will know anyway, based on your appearance or a simple monitoring of your cholesterol level or blood pressure. If you haven't been doing what was suggested, from taking a new medication to changing your diet or beginning an exercise routine, just be honest about it.

Have you tried a new diet but failed? Is your prescribed pill literally too big to swallow? Is your new medication upsetting your stomach? Let your doctors know.

By having open and honest dialogues with your doctors, you're more likely to come up with solutions that might be more manageable for you, or you can agree to try again and talk about specific ways to combat your challenges, so you can be more compliant and make changes to improve your health.

Complying with your doctor's recommendations is how you hold up your end of the bargain.

Fibbing to your doctors — or worse yet, blaming your doctor for your own inadequacies of compliance — will get you nowhere. Take responsibility for your own actions. Fess up.

Complying with your doctor's recommendations is how you hold up your end of the bargain. It's how you take responsibility for the part you play on your health care team. From little things your doctor might suggest, such as taking a pill with a meal, to bigger changes like becoming more physically active or choosing healthier foods, you are receiving directions that may enhance the quality of your life.

The success of your treatment is, of course, likely to be highest when you comply with these recommendations. This is both good news and bad news. The bad news is that while compliance gives you your best chance at good health, it can often be challenging. It's not easy to change your lifestyle habits or to remember to take medications as directed, but the good news is that you are the primary person in control. Positive changes are possible if you're willing to put forth the effort to make them.

After each visit, take a few minutes to write down how you will follow through, what tests are being set up, any prescriptions you need to fill, and anything else that needs to be scheduled.

Tool 11: Post-Visit Action Plan

Break down your doctor's suggestions from **Tool 5: Health Care Visit** into realistic, manageable actions you can take each day toward improving your health, and write the actions on **Tool 11: Post-Visit Action Plan**.

Post-Visit Action Plan

Name _____ Doctor's Name _____ Date ____ / ____ / ____

Steps to take in diet

1. _____

2. _____

3. _____

4. _____

Steps to take in exercise

1. _____

2. _____

3. _____

4. _____

Steps to take in lifestyle modifications

1. _____

2. _____

3. _____

4. _____

Steps to take with medications

1. _____

2. _____

3. _____

4. _____

Notes _____

Referrals _____

Chapter 7: Taking Alternative Routes

Sometimes you want to go beyond your doctor's recommendations, try another approach, or get a second opinion. Remember you are taking care of your body, and it's okay to explore your options.

After my first cognitive impairment exams in 2012, a doctor at a major medical center gave me the official (scary) diagnosis of Early Stage Alzheimer's disease. Even though I knew my memory was slipping, this diagnosis was disturbing. It was huge. It was life altering. And I didn't feel comfortable just going with it.

I was prescribed a medication to help slow down the decline of my memory, but I couldn't bring myself to get it filled. I couldn't explain why. Something just didn't feel right.

After debating what to do, I went with my gut feeling and decided to get a second opinion. My primary care doctor referred me to a second neurologist, and I underwent a second neurological and psychological exam.

"Draw a clock," the new neurologist instructed.

I drew a circle and wrote the number 12 where the 4 should go, which messed me up from the get-go. Gail's mouth dropped. I looked at her and shook my head, too befuddled to go any further.

The neurologist then wrote the number 12 at the top of the clock, which prompted me to remember where the rest of the numbers should go.

I filled in the clock, but was immediately stopped again by her next request.

"Please draw the time as 10 after 11," she said.

Ten after 11 made no sense to me; I couldn't remember where to put the long hand or the short hand.

After completing my exam, it turned out that my new neurologist agreed with my initial diagnosis.

"But," she added, "I believe you're much worse than what you were told. And you need to be on two medications, not just one."

I filled the two prescriptions immediately and to this day have been fully compliant with her treatment plan. As a result of the medications she prescribed, my family and I immediately noticed a marked improvement in my memory.

Perhaps my condition had worsened during my time without treatment. Then again, maybe the second exam uncovered more than the first. I'll never know, but what I do know is that I'm glad I did both.

Sometimes, even when we do all the right things: prepare for the doctor, relay our information, and make sure to get all our questions answered, things can still feel wrong. You can still end up frustrated, angry, or doubting.

Go ahead and get a second opinion if you feel you need it. If it's possible to go somewhere else, do it. It may take time and add to your costs, but your health — your life — is worth it if you feel uncomfortable for any reason, even if like me, you can't explain why. Before choosing another doctor, you may want to solicit advice and suggestions from friends and family, but be sure to do your own research before making a decision.

With the vast amount of information available today, a natural thought is to search the Internet. Reputable sites and trusted news sources can educate you on symptoms, diagnoses, and treatments. Visit well-known sites like Mayo

Clinic and government sites for the most accurate, up-to-date statistics and information. And don't believe everything you read. Often, you'll find information that hasn't been updated for years or people sharing widely varying opinions based on their own experiences. Do your homework and go with what feels right for you.

Remember that you have the option to research any treatment, drug or surgery that's recommended to you. Medicine is an art as well as a science. There may be one diagnosis, but there are multiple ways to treat it.

When diagnosed with a chronic or life-threatening illness, you may also choose to seek out psychological or religious guidance to help you manage emotionally as well as physically.

Don't let resentment or any thought of a stigma keep you from the benefits of talking to a professional listener.

Two years after the life-threatening illness that landed me in the hospital for two weeks afraid to go to sleep, I came to terms with the fact that I had to choose between my successful dental career and my life. It was devastating to give up the practice I had built and to resign from my position as Assistant Professor of Prosthodontics at Harvard School of Dental Medicine. I turned to counseling to help me through the transition and grief I felt.

For the next 10 years, I received monthly disability insurance payments because of my debilitating condition. When I was forced, at the 10-year mark, to justify my disability in order to continue receiving payments, I sought counseling again. This time, to manage the tragic injustice I felt.

After a particularly painful back surgery in 2010, when I was left with no follow-up care, I sought counseling to manage my pain, and shortly afterward to deal with my cognitive impairment from Alzheimer's.

Each counselor helped by listening to me, validating me, and teaching me methods to help me live a more proactive life. In each situation, the counseling was beneficial.

While referring a patient to a counselor can be a fallback for some doctors who want to suggest that your ailments are "all in your head," it is sometimes wise to explore this avenue even if you don't feel that is the case. Your brain controls everything in your body, yet it is often overlooked. Don't let resentment or any thought of a stigma keep you from the benefits of talking to a professional listener. Even if you are emotionally "normal," your physical troubles might be causing emotional distress, and a counselor can help you cope.

While you may have the support of family and friends, they may not want to hear about your illness for their own reasons, or they may offer advice you neither want nor need. Often, you'll find yourself alone with your thoughts, and if those thoughts start careening toward a ditch, it might help to let a counselor hear what you're telling yourself. An objective listener can be beneficial, and simply listening to yourself say out loud what you've been saying in your head can be eye opening.

Other options of support include following a reputable medical blog, where you can get expert information and advice, or joining a support group, either in person or online. With people connecting like never before, you may find someone who can exactly relate to what you are going through, or who has been there and found ways to cope, or who can simply sympathize with your thoughts and feelings.

Chapter 8: Preparing for Tests, Procedures & Surgeries

As you can see by my Body Chart at the end of the book, I am no stranger to medical tests, procedures, and surgeries.

In the past three years alone, I've been tested for balance disorder, my driving abilities in light of my cognitive problems, to rule out sleep apnea, and to determine the cause of my stomach discomfort.

I've had MRIs and CT scans on everything from my heart to my gall bladder to my prostate. In my lifetime, I've had three back surgeries, hand surgery for sliced tendons, gall-bladder surgery and prostate surgery. I've endured endoscopies, colonoscopies, pulmonary function tests, and more.

Preparing the paperwork you'll take with you for a medical test, procedure, or surgery is really no different than preparing for an office visit. You should still plan to be armed with **Tool 2: Current Medications, Tool 3: Current Physicians & Health Care Providers, Tool 5: Health Care Visit** (if you have last-minute questions to ask before the test, procedure, or surgery), **Tool 7: Personal Health History, Tool 8: Family Health History, Tool 9: Current Symptoms Body Chart**. The same questions that are on these tools will likely be asked of you in person or on office forms. Remember to bring a copy for yourself and a copy for your doctor.

Tool 12: Checklist for Tests, Procedures & Surgeries

Be sure your medication list is up to date with not only the medications, but also the dosage you take each day and how often you take it. Use **Tool 12: Checklist for Tests, Procedures & Surgeries** to help you prepare in other ways.

In the event of a hospital stay, it's important for you to take along all essential prescribed medications in their original bottles. The doctors and nursing staff may not want you to keep them with you because they will want to know, and legally must know, what you're taking and when you're taking it. In many cases, however, it can take a day or more for a hospital to establish your medication regimen. It takes time to get the doctor's order, the insurance company's approval, and for a hospital's pharmacy to fill the prescriptions. During this time, you will want to have your own medications as a backup, for both your physical well-being and your peace of mind.

Upon discharge from a hospital, ask for a day's worth of medications so you won't have to stop on the way home.

During one of my many overnight stays, the hospital staff was unable to obtain several of the medications I was routinely taking. I called Gail, and she immediately brought over the needed medications, nearly a dozen bottles. The nurse labeled each with my name, put them in a locked cabinet in the nurses' station. She then gave them to me as prescribed by my doctor. This arrangement was beneficial for us both.

Tool 13: Daily Medications

If you take your medications with you, you will also want to bring a list of what you take and when. **Tool 2: Current Medications** will suffice. But if you'd like to simplify it, you may want to use **Tool 13: Daily Medications**. Gail and I also find this tool essential for our daily use at home.

Upon discharge from a procedure or a hospital, ask for any prescriptions you might need, and see if you can get a day's worth of the medications so you won't have to stop at a pharmacy on your way home. No matter what time the nurse says you might be discharged, it is typically a lengthy process, and once you are out, you won't want to delay getting home.

Tool 14: Medication Refills

When you get a new medication, it's important to note the refill date, so you won't be caught off guard and in need of your essential medications. **Tool 14: Medication Refills** is an easy way to keep track of the dates you will need to call in or when you might need to see a doctor, if an office visit is required for a renewal.

Five Wishes

One last thing to do before any procedure or surgery is to let your final wishes be known. Often this comes up as we age or become especially ill. Don't wait until then to decide what you'd like to do. An extraordinary tool that can aid you in answering questions about your final wishes is not one I created, but one I have used and feel is important. It's called Five Wishes and can be found at **www.agingwithdignity.org**.

Visit the site to learn how you can let your doctors and family know the person you would like to make your health care decisions if you can't make them. You can also let them know other things, such as what kind of medical treatment you would like or not like, how comfortable you would like to be kept, and how you would like people to treat you.

The website has documents you can personalize and print. Five Wishes currently meets legal requirements in 42 states and is useful in all of them. [1]

---

[1] www.agingwithdignity.org/five-wishes.php

Checklist for Tests, Procedures & Surgeries

Before any test or procedure:

____ Check with your insurance company for pre-approval and co-payment information

____ Ask if there's a payment plan, if needed

____ Be compliant with the instructions you're given before your test, procedure, or surgery

Bring:

____ Tool 2: Current Medications

____ Tool 3: Current Physicians & Health Care Providers

____ Tool 5: Health Care Visit

____ Tool 7: Personal Health History

____ Tool 8: Family Health History

____ Tool 9: Current Symptoms Body Chart

____ Any requested office paperwork

Other items you may want to bring:

____ Essential medications

____ Toothbrush/toothpaste

____ Socks/slippers

____ Pajamas/robe

____ An extra blanket

____ Comfort items (your phone, laptop, iPad, music, books, magazines, etc.)

____ Earplugs/earphones

____ Phone/laptop power cord and possibly an extension cord (so your electronics can reach your bed)

____ Bottled water/snack bars

____ Shampoo/conditioner

____ Lotion

Be prepared:

____ Arrive 30 minutes before your appointment, so you'll feel more relaxed and can fill out any additional forms

____ Expect to wait; bring items with you to pass the time

____ Have a driver, if recommended

After the test, procedure, or surgery:

____ Ask what to do if there are complications

____ Ask about any questions you have about medications, pain relievers or precautions

Once you're home:

____ Read and comply with post-procedure instruction, know possible side effects and what to watch for

Daily Medications

Name _____ Date _____ / _____ / _____

Medication Rx #	Daily Dosage	List in order taken during the day			
		AM	Noon	PM	Bedtime
Medication Name here *Rx # here* *You may want to highlight those that are essential* *and not highlight those that are optional.*					

Medication Refills

Name _____ Date _____ / _____ / _____

Medication Rx #	June		July		August		September	
	Refill Date	Check Off	Refill Date	Check Off	Refill Date	Check Off	Refill Date	Check Off
Medication Name here *Rx # here*	6/13		7/13		8/13		9/13	

Chapter 9: Checking Your Insurance Coverage

Several years ago, I underwent a sleep study to test for sleep apnea. Prior to my appointment at the major medical center where the test would be conducted, I met with my doctor, who let me know a device would arrive in the mail for me to use prior to the study. Sure enough, I received what looked like a sophisticated watch, with instructions that said to wear it 24 hours a day for the seven days leading up to the study.

The device was used to determine my natural sleep patterns in my home environment before they monitored my sleep at the center. I was instructed to keep it on until I arrived there. Simple enough.

I complied with the directions and when the time came, I completed the overnight sleep study at the center. About a month after the study, which had been pre-approved by my insurance company, I got an invoice in the mail for $1,500.

To my shock, I had been billed for the rental payment of the device!

It turned out the staff at the center had requested pre-approval for the device from my insurance company, but it was denied because the insurance company considered it experimental. We, however, were never told of this.

We complained and appealed, but ultimately were successful only in arranging a payment plan, which still left us responsible for the entire amount.

Expensive lesson learned.

Prior to any tests, procedures or surgeries, find out exactly what will be covered. Typically, our only thought about insurance is making the monthly payment. It's not until we have a claim that we read what our policy actually covers, and it's often too little, too late.

In most cases, the office staff will call your insurance company for pre-approvals, but that doesn't always mean that everything will be approved or that everything will be fully covered. Don't be caught unaware. Be prepared.

Ask the office staff what you are going to owe when all is said and done. Read your policy. Know your co-payments and deductibles.

Should you receive an unexpected bill, immediately contact your doctor's office and insurance company. Often, mistakes are made or coverage is delayed because of miscommunication. These discrepancies typically can be resolved over the phone.

Tool 15: Communication Log

 In the meantime, keep track of your conversations with your insurance company and those billing you with **Tool 15: Communication Log**. It's essential for you to get the name of each person you speak with, and jot down what was said and what the next step will be. Also make a note of anything you need to do to follow up, and be sure to note the date and time of the call.

Phone conversations typically are recorded and documented by insurance companies, but your own meticulous record will be your greatest ally. It will help you follow up and keep the facts straight.

Clearing up a discrepancy can take several phone calls and lots of time. Documenting the details will help you through until you reach a resolution. Don't give up.

To make your calls the most productive, ask these important questions:

- Will someone call me back?

- Who will call me and when?

- If I don't receive a call, who should I contact and at what number?

- Ask them to repeat any needed information, so you can accurately document it.

Communication Log

Date	Name of person I spoke to	What was said	What the follow up will be	Action I need to take

Chapter 10: Assembling Your Support Team

Sometimes, you are too sick to do things for yourself, and you have to rely on others to step in on your behalf.

A few years ago, while Gail and I were in the midst of managing my cognitive condition as well as various other health issues, Gail was diagnosed with uterine cancer. The tables turned, and I became her primary caregiver.

My role increased significantly when we later learned that the uterine cancer had metastasized to one of her lungs. She underwent surgery to remove a tumor and the lobe of her lung where the cancer had grown, but during her post-op recovery, the seriousness of her condition increased as she found it difficult to eat or drink anything without being thrown into a terrible, prolonged coughing spell. Her voice went hoarse, and her breathing and swallowing became more difficult.

Gail saw specialist after specialist, hoping one of them would be able to provide an answer as to why she had developed this chronic cough and why her health was continuing to deteriorate.

After a couple months of making the rounds, and wishing and hoping and expecting things to get better, I called her pulmonary doctor to try to get an appointment that I was determined would result in her re-admission to a hospital. It was a Friday, and I knew that if we didn't reach the doctor and get her admitted by the end of the day, we'd have to wait out the weekend. That was a risk I didn't want to take. As a close observer of Gail's health for more than 40 years, I knew how desperately ill she was, and I felt deeply compelled to take immediate, assertive action.

I discovered her doctor was out of town, and I was frustrated when it seemed impossible to get an appointment with any other doctor in his practice. I was fed up with waiting for return phone calls and getting nowhere.

I was out of ideas.

That night as I was lying awake in bed — possibly delirious from lack of sleep and most certainly pumped up on the adrenaline from feeling frantic — it popped into my head to try to contact her doctor by email. So what if he was out of town? If he was the only doctor who could admit her, then he was the one I needed to reach.

I hopped out of bed, plunked down in our office chair and sat in the dark staring at my computer screen. I willed the right words to come to me despite my cognitive disorder. In my email, I outlined her symptoms and relayed the details of her severe daily distress. I pleaded for her admission to the hospital, where she could receive a comprehensive evaluation and get a diagnosis from her team of physicians; I wanted them to come to her.

I wrote: "For me and my family to literally run around for the next two to three months, from doc to doc, and from test to test, seeking a diagnosis, treatment plan, and treatments would be totally inappropriate. Her hospitalization would give the team of physicians the opportunity to best communicate and consult with one another efficiently and effectively. I am asking for your help from the depth of my heart to admit Gail immediately. Help, help, help is all I can say."

I guessed at the doctor's email address, trying multiple combinations of his name and practice, until I hit on one that didn't come back as undeliverable. I fired off the email at 3:39 a.m. with the subject line: URGENT. It was now Saturday morning, officially the weekend.

When I woke up five hours later, I checked my inbox. There was no reply. Though it was irrational to have expected an answer so quickly, especially when I could have only hoped I'd actually reached the doctor, I knew we didn't have any time to lose.

I immediately forwarded the email to the only other person I could think of who might be able to help us: Gail's surgeon. He was not currently treating her, but he had previously given us his email address. He responded immediately. And not by email, but the old-fashioned way: by calling me. I was elated.

One day, you might find yourself in need of assistance. Take time now to list people you think will support you.

Gail was admitted that afternoon — as soon as the surgeon could get a room for her — and she remained in the hospital for an entire week. A feeding tube was placed in her stomach so she would no longer have to eat and drink fluids, and her lungs could get a rest from the coughing. Finally, she was receiving the care she so desperately needed. I will be forever thankful for her surgeon's quick response to our needs, and I am so glad I pressed the issue.

Just as I was there for Gail, she of course has been there for me countless times. Many years ago, when I was not acting as my own best health care advocate, and I did not have my charts and list of symptoms and medications, I dreaded every doctor appointment. I especially dreaded visiting new doctors because it was both exhausting and depressing to explain my entire health history over and over again.

At one of my lowest points, before my chronic bronchial infections were diagnosed, Gail stepped in on my behalf. In her search for remedies for my condition, she came across a doctor she felt might be able to help, and made an appointment for me. Because I had been through this routine so many times before, I put my foot down and refused to go. As my advocate, she went without me — by herself, to my appointment. She went to tell my story for me and to spare me from any further exhaustion or disappointment. If ever it was the thought that counted, that was it. When the time came that I could look back on what she did for my benefit, I was so appreciative of her depth of understanding and so amazed at the support she showed.

Tool 16: Assembling Your Support Team

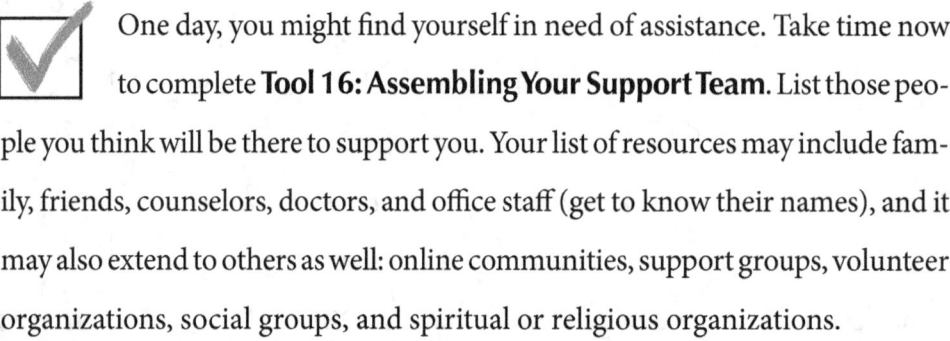 One day, you might find yourself in need of assistance. Take time now to complete **Tool 16: Assembling Your Support Team.** List those people you think will be there to support you. Your list of resources may include family, friends, counselors, doctors, and office staff (get to know their names), and it may also extend to others as well: online communities, support groups, volunteer organizations, social groups, and spiritual or religious organizations.

Facing a medical challenge and its accompanying symptoms can be emotionally devastating, whether you are the patient or the caregiver. Keep a copy of **Tool 16: Assembling Your Support Team** to use as a quick reference and to remind yourself of people and organizations you can turn to.

If you aren't currently facing a medical challenge, you have the advantage of compiling your list while you're well. It's helpful to have this list of names and numbers ready for yourself and your loved ones, especially in case of emergency.

From my own experience, I can tell you that sometimes your biggest allies will be exactly those people you expected, but sometimes they won't be. Sometimes, you'll get help from those you least expected it from and vice versa.

If offers of help don't come from those you were counting on, try not to take it personally. Not all of your friends and family may recognize your needs or be able to help as you'd like. As much as possible, be prepared for this and try to adjust. And don't be afraid to ask for assistance. Some people simply don't know how they can help.

Acknowledge the support you do receive. It may come in the form of a phone call or a dinner. It may be emotional support, financial, or social. Whatever it is, say, "Thank you," and be grateful.

As my cognitive condition progresses, I know I will be relying more and more on those around me to speak for me and manage my affairs. I am confident that the information on my charts and in my histories will help them answer questions and best prepare me for my doctors' appointments. They will also help me to remember what I most want to say and help my doctors do their best work on my behalf.

Acknowledge the support you do receive. Say, "Thank you," and be grateful.

Fill out the tools in this book and use them to spare both yourself and your loved ones from having to remember, relive, and relay the same information over and over. Use them to help you prepare, help you explain, keep you on track, keep you connected, and help you to put your best foot forward so you can receive the validation, care, and support you need and deserve.

Do all you can — and you can do a lot starting right here — to make your health and your life the best it can be.

I wish you well.

My Support Team

Name	Phone	Email

Tools You Can Use

To download copies online,
visit www.EnhanceYourHealthCare.com

Enter 2ZGY8FL7 to access forms.

Tools You Can Use

Current Symptoms

Patient Name _____ Date _____ / _____ / _____

Head/Mental
____ Anxiety
____ Depression
____ Memory loss (long-term)
____ Memory loss (short-term)
____ Mood swings
____ Nervousness
____ Other _____

Head/Physical
____ Dizziness
____ Headaches
____ Redness in the face
____ Seizures
____ Other _____

Eyes
____ Bloody
____ Blurry vision
____ Change in vision
____ Double vision
____ Dryness
____ Floaters in eye
____ Infection
____ Itchy
____ Night blindness
____ Pain
____ Redness
____ Sensitivity to light
____ Other _____

Heart
____ Fluttering (skipping beats)
____ Pain
____ Pressure
____ Rapid heartbeat
____ Other _____

Nose
____ Bleeding
____ Dripping
____ Dryness
____ Frequent colds
____ Sneezing
____ Stuffiness
____ Other _____

Ears
____ Bleeding
____ Discharge
____ Frequent ear infections
____ Hearing problems
____ Pain
____ Redness
____ Ringing in ears
____ Waxy
____ Other _____

Mouth
____ Bad breath
____ Bleeding gums
____ Cold sores
____ Dental pain
____ Discomfort in jaw joint
____ Dryness
____ Excess saliva
____ Infection
____ Loose teeth
____ Sensitive teeth (hot/cold)
____ Sores that don't heal
____ White sores
____ Other _____

Neck
____ Neck pain/stiffness
____ Swollen lymph nodes
____ Other _____

Throat
____ Dryness
____ Difficulty swallowing
____ Difficulty speaking
____ Excessive clearing of throat
____ Frequent sore throats
____ Hoarseness
____ Mucus
____ Other _____

Chest/Breast/Lungs
____ Coughing
____ Coughing up blood
____ Coughing up mucus
____ Discolored mucus
____ Frequent colds
____ Pain or discomfort
____ Shortness of breath
____ Unusual discharge
____ Other _____

Back
____ Aches
____ Cramps
____ Pain
____ Other _____

Shoulders/Arms/Elbows/Hands
____ Numbness
____ Pain
____ Swelling
____ Tingling
____ Other _____

Allergies

_____

_____

Current Symptoms

Patient Name _____ Date _____ / _____ / _____

Legs/Knees
____ Cramps
____ Pain
____ Swelling
____ Tingling
____ Other _____

Ankles/Feet
____ Burning
____ Dryness
____ Flaking
____ Itchy
____ Numbness
____ Pain
____ Sores that won't heal
____ Swelling
____ Toe pain
____ Other _____

Skin
____ Dryness
____ Hives
____ Itchy
____ Moles that changed color
____ Rashes
____ Sores
____ Sores that don't heal

Urinary Tract
____ Blood in urine
____ Burning/painful urination
____ Difficulty urinating
____ Frequent urinary infections
____ Frequent urination
____ Incontinence
____ Other

Nails
____ Brittle
____ Change in color
____ Fungus
____ Other _____

Gastrointestinal
____ Abdominal pain
____ Blood in stool
____ Change in bowels
____ Constipation
____ Diarrhea
____ Heartburn
____ Hemorrhoids
____ Nausea
____ Poor appetite
____ Reflux
____ Tarry stool
____ Vomiting
____ Vomiting up blood
____ Other _____

Reproductive System
____ Bleeding
____ Change in flow
____ Irregular menstrual cycle
____ No periods
____ Pain
____ Staining
____ Testicular pain
____ Unusual discharge
____ Other _____

General
____ Anemia
____ Difficulty balancing
____ Dizziness
____ Easy bruising or bleeding
____ Excessive sweating

____ Excessive thirst
____ Fainting
____ Fatigue
____ Fevers/chills
____ Frequent urination
____ Heat or cold intolerance
____ Hot flashes
____ Involuntary movements
____ Joint pain
____ Lightheaded
____ Limited range of motion
____ Muscular pain
____ Need to sleep upright
____ Numbness
____ Pain
____ Recent weight gain
____ Recent weight loss
____ Shortness of breath/rest
____ Shortness of breath/exertion
____ Swollen glands
____ Trauma to a specific area
____ Tremors
____ Trouble sleeping
____ Weakness
____ Other _____

On a scale of 1-10 (1 is lowest, 10 is highest), rate your current level of pain for each symptom.

_____

_____

_____

_____

Current Medications

Patient Name _____   Date _____ / _____ / _____

Medication Name Rx #	Dosage Times/Day	When Taken	Prescribing Doctor	Reason for Taking	Notes/Side Effects/Allergies

Current Medications, Tool 2

Current Physicians & Health Care Providers

Patient Name _____ Date _____ / _____ / _____

Doctor's Name: _____ Specialty: _____

Address: _____ Phone Number: _____

Doctor's Name: _____ Specialty: _____

Address: _____ Phone Number: _____

Doctor's Name: _____ Specialty: _____

Address: _____ Phone Number: _____

Doctor's Name: _____ Specialty: _____

Address: _____ Phone Number: _____

Doctor's Name: _____ Specialty: _____

Address: _____ Phone Number: _____

Doctor's Name: _____ Specialty: _____

Address: _____ Phone Number: _____

Doctor's Name: _____ Specialty: _____

Address: _____ Phone Number: _____

Doctor's Name: _____ Specialty: _____

Address: _____ Phone Number: _____

My Personal Top 10 List

Name _____   Date _____ / _____ / _____

Three things I love to do but haven't done in more than a year

1. _____

2. _____

3. _____

Pick one and do it this month.

If I were invisible for a day, where would I go and what would I do?

4. _____

Consider going there and doing that.

Three friends I would love to spend the day with

5. _____

6. _____

7. _____

Call or write them and choose one day to spend with each, or get them all together.

Three things I loved to do as a kid

8. _____

9. _____

10. _____

Do them now.

Health Care Visit

Patient Name _____   Appt. Date ___ / ___ / ___

Name of Health Care Provider _____   Appt. Time _____

Address _____   Phone _____

Top Concerns
1.
Notes/Recommendations:
2.
Notes/Recommendations:
3.
Notes/Recommendations:
4.
Notes/Recommendations:
5.
Notes/Recommendations:
Conclusions/Follow-up needed:

Health Care Visit

Name _____ Doctor's Name _____ Date ____ / ____ / ____

Diet _____

_____

_____

Exercise _____

_____

_____

Lifestyle modifications (Sleep, stress reduction, etc.) _____

_____

_____

Medications (What to take, dosage, when and how long to take it, side effects, managing side effects)

_____

_____

Call doctor if _____

_____

_____

When to schedule next appointment _____

Referrals _____

_____

Additional notes _____

_____

_____

_____

Typical Daily Symptoms

Name _____   Date _____ / _____ / _____

Time	Symptoms	Notes
5-6 a.m.		
6-7 a.m.		
7-8 a.m.		
8-9 a.m.		
9-10 a.m.		
10-11 a.m.		
11 a-12 p		
12-1 p.m.		
1-2 p.m.		
2-3 p.m.		
3-4 p.m.		
4-5 p.m.		
5-6 p.m.		
6-7 p.m.		
7-8 p.m.		
8-9 p.m.		
9-10 p.m.		
10-11 p.m.		
11-12 p.m.		
12 p -3 a		
3-4 a.m.		
4-5 a.m.		

Personal Health History

Patient Name _____ Date _____ / _____ / _____

Previous and Current Conditions

Year condition began (and ended, if applicable)

_____ Allergies	_____ Hearing loss	_____ Obesity
_____ Alzheimer's disease	_____ Heartburn	_____ Osteopenia
_____ Anemia	_____ Heart disease	_____ Osteoporosis
_____ Arthritis	_____ Hernia	_____ Pacemaker
_____ Anxiety	_____ High blood pressure	_____ Parkinson's disease
_____ Asthma	_____ HIV	_____ Pelvic pain
_____ Back pain	_____ Incontinence	_____ Pregnancy difficulties
_____ Blood disease	_____ Infection	_____ Respiratory problems
_____ Cancer	_____ Staph infection	_____ Sciatica
_____ Cataract	_____ Infertility problems	_____ Seizures
_____ Chemical dependency	_____ Joint problems	_____ Shingles
_____ Circulation problems	_____ Joint replacement	_____ Sleep difficulties
_____ Constipation	_____ Kidney problems	_____ Swelling
_____ Depression	_____ Liver problems	_____ Thyroid problems
_____ Diabetes	_____ Memory loss (long-term)	_____ Tooth sensitivity
_____ Emphysema	_____ Memory loss (short-term)	_____ Tuberculosis
_____ Emotional disorders	_____ Mental illness	_____ Vision problems
_____ Fractures	_____ Migraines	_____ Weakness
_____ Genital disease	_____ Miscarriage	_____ Weight gain (significant)
_____ Glaucoma	_____ Multiple sclerosis	_____ Weight loss (significant)
_____ Headaches	_____ Numbness	_____ Other _____

Injury History

Injury _____	Year _____	Injury _____	Year _____
Injury _____	Year _____	Injury _____	Year _____
Injury _____	Year _____	Injury _____	Year _____

Surgery History

Surgery _____	Year _____	Surgery _____	Year _____
Surgery _____	Year _____	Surgery _____	Year _____
Surgery _____	Year _____	Surgery _____	Year _____

Personal Health History

Patient Name _____ Date _____ / _____ / _____

Chronological list of allergies, conditions, injuries, surgeries, etc.	**Age**	**Approximate date**
_____	_____	_____
_____	_____	_____
_____	_____	_____
_____	_____	_____
_____	_____	_____
_____	_____	_____
_____	_____	_____
_____	_____	_____
_____	_____	_____
_____	_____	_____
_____	_____	_____
_____	_____	_____
_____	_____	_____
_____	_____	_____
_____	_____	_____
_____	_____	_____
_____	_____	_____
_____	_____	_____
_____	_____	_____

Family Health History

Patient Name _____ Date _____ / _____ / _____

_____ Anemia	_____ Glaucoma	_____ Obesity
_____ Allergies	_____ Headaches	_____ Osteopenia
_____ Alzheimer's disease	_____ Hearing loss	_____ Osteoporosis
_____ Arthritis	_____ Heart condition	_____ Pacemaker
_____ Asthma	_____ Heart disease	_____ Parkinson's disease
_____ Anxiety	_____ High blood pressure	_____ Pregnancy difficulties
_____ Back Pain	_____ HIV	_____ Respiratory problems
_____ Blood Disease	_____ Staph infections	_____ Sciatica
_____ Cancer	_____ Joint problems	_____ Seizures
_____ Cataract	_____ Joint replacement	_____ Shingles
_____ Chemical dependency	_____ Kidney problems	_____ Sleep Difficulties
_____ Circulation problems	_____ Liver problems	_____ Thyroid problems
_____ Depression	_____ Memory loss (long-term)	_____ Tuberculosis
_____ Diabetes	_____ Memory loss (short-term)	_____ Vision problems
_____ Emotional disorders	_____ Mental illness	_____ Weight gain (significant)
_____ Emphysema	_____ Miscarriage	_____ Weight Loss (significant)
_____ Genital disease	_____ Multiple sclerosis	_____ Other _____

Notes _____

_____

_____

_____

_____

On the back, write your family health history according to the family members affected.
Having this list in both forms gives you easy references depending on the way you're asked for the information.

Family Member	Full Name	Age	Health Status	Cause of death/age, if applicable
Mother				
Maternal grandmother				
Maternal grandfather				
Aunts, uncles, cousins with notable conditions				
Father				
Paternal grandmother				
Paternal grandfather				
Aunts, uncles, cousins with notable conditions				
My siblings				

Current Symptoms

Patient Name _____ Date _____

My Front Left Side

My Front Right Side

Current Symptoms Body Chart, Tool 9 — 1 of 2

Current Symptoms

Patient Name _____ Date _____

My Back Left Side

My Back Right Side

_____
_____
_____
_____
_____
_____
_____
_____
_____
_____
_____
_____
_____
_____
_____
_____
_____
_____
_____
_____
_____

_____
_____
_____
_____
_____
_____
_____
_____
_____
_____
_____
_____
_____
_____
_____
_____
_____
_____
_____
_____

Evaluation Form (Office Visit)

Doctor's Name _____ Appt. Date ____ / ____ / ____

Address _____ Specialty _____

Rating the Office Visit				
Reception				
1. How many minutes I waited to be seen	0-15 mins.	15-30 mins.	30-45 mins.	45+ mins.
2. How many minutes I waited once in the room	0-15 mins.	15-30 mins.	30-45 mins.	45+ mins.
1= Disagree, 2 = Somewhat agree, 3 = Agree, 4 = Strongly agree				
3. I was warmly greeted by the staff.	1	2	3	4
4. I was warmly greeted by the doctor.	1	2	3	4
5. The doctor respectfully accepted my prepared forms.	1	2	3	4
6. The doctor paid attention to my medical issue(s).	1	2	3	4
7. The doctor addressed my top concerns.	1	2	3	4
8. The doctor validated my medical concerns.	1	2	3	4
Communication Skills				
1= Inadequate, 2= Adequate, 3 = Better than average, 4 = Excellent				
1. Listened attentively	1	2	3	4
2. Seemed caring and compassionate	1	2	3	4
3. Exhibited acceptable "bedside manner"	1	2	3	4
4. Answered all my questions appropriately	1	2	3	4
5. Interacted well with office staff	1	2	3	4
6. Treated my family/friends well	1	2	3	4
Clinical Skills				
1= Inadequate, 2= Adequate, 3 = Better than average, 4 = Excellent				
1. Spent an adequate amount of time with me	1	2	3	4
2. Quality of the clinical examination	1	2	3	4
3. Management of my medical issues	1	2	3	4
4. Diagnostic skills and clinical judgment	1	2	3	4
5. Made appropriate referrals, if needed	1	2	3	4
Will you see this doctor again? Yes No (If no, keep this for records in case you are referred in the future.)				
If not, why not?				
Comments regarding office staff:				
Additional comments:				

Evaluation Form (Myself)

Doctor's Name _____ Appt. Date ____ / ____ / ____

Address _____ Specialty _____

Rating Myself		
Preparation		
1. Time of appointment:		
2. Time I arrived:		
3. Completed paperwork prior to visit, if requested	Yes	No
4. Arrived early to fill out paperwork, if needed	Yes	No
5. Complied with all preparation requests prior to visit	Yes	No
6. Brought completed Tool 1: Current Symptoms	Yes	No
7. Brought completed Tool 2: Current Medications	Yes	No
8. Brought completed Tool 3: Current Physicians & Health Care Providers	Yes	No
9. Brought completed Tool 5: Health Care Visit	Yes	No
10. Brought completed Tool 6: Typical Daily Symptoms	Yes	No
11. Brought completed Tool 7: Personal Health History	Yes	No
12. Brought completed Tool 8: Family Health History	Yes	No
13. Brought completed Tool 9: Current Symptoms Body Chart	Yes	No
14. Brought completed Tool 12: Checklist for Tests, Procedures & Surgeries, if needed	Yes	No
15. Brought completed Tool 13: Daily Medications, if needed	Yes	No
At the Visit		
1. Communicated effectively with the staff	Yes	No
2. Gave doctor/staff a copy of my tool(s)	Yes	No
3. Voiced each concern	Yes	No
4. Completed front Tool 5: Health Care Visit	Yes	No
5. Made follow-up appointment, if needed	Yes	No
After the Visit		
1. Completed Tool 10: Evaluation of Office Visit	Yes	No
2. Completed back of Tool 5: Health Care Visit	Yes	No
3. Completed Tool 11: Post-Visit Action Plan	Yes	No
What I could have done differently to make the appointment more productive:		

Post-Visit Action Plan

Name _____ Doctor's Name _____ Date ____ / ____ / ____

Steps to take in diet

1. _____
2. _____
3. _____
4. _____

Steps to take in exercise

1. _____
2. _____
3. _____
4. _____

Steps to take in lifestyle modifications

1. _____
2. _____
3. _____
4. _____

Steps to take with medications

1. _____
2. _____
3. _____
4. _____

Notes _____

Referrals _____

Checklist for Tests, Procedures & Surgeries

Before any test or procedure:

____ Check with your insurance company for pre-approval and co-payment information

____ Ask if there's a payment plan, if needed

____ Be compliant with the instructions you're given before your test, procedure, or surgery

Bring:

____ Tool 2: Current Medications

____ Tool 3: Current Physicians & Health Care Providers

____ Tool 5: Health Care Visit

____ Tool 7: Personal Health History

____ Tool 8: Family Health History

____ Tool 9: Current Symptoms Body Chart

____ Any requested office paperwork

Other items you may want to bring:

____ Essential medications

____ Toothbrush/toothpaste

____ Socks/slippers

____ Pajamas/robe

____ An extra blanket

____ Comfort items (your phone, laptop, iPad, music, books, magazines, etc.)

____ Earplugs/earphones

____ Phone/laptop power cord and possibly an extension cord (so your electronics can reach your bed)

____ Bottled water/snack bars

____ Shampoo/conditioner

____ Lotion

Be prepared:

____ Arrive 30 minutes before your appointment, so you'll feel more relaxed and can fill out any additional forms

____ Expect to wait; bring items with you to pass the time

____ Have a driver, if recommended

After the test, procedure, or surgery:

____ Ask what to do if there are complications

____ Ask about any questions you have about medications, pain relievers or precautions

Once you're home:

____ Read and comply with post-procedure instruction, know possible side effects and what to watch for

Daily Medications

Name _____   Date _____ / _____ / _____

Medication Rx #	Daily Dosage	List in order taken during the day			
		AM	Noon	PM	Bedtime

Medication Refills

Name _____ Date _____ / _____ / _____

Medication Rx #	June		July		August		September	
	Refill Date	Check Off	Refill Date	Check Off	Refill Date	Check Off	Refill Date	Check Off

Communication Log

Date	Name of person I spoke to	What was said	What the follow up will be	Action I need to take

My Support Team

Name	Phone	Email

About the Authors

Alexander "Sandy" Halperin, DDS, was born and raised in Springfield, Massachusetts. After receiving his dental degree from New York University College of Dentistry and his specialty training in prosthodontics at Eastman Dental Center in Rochester, New York, he enjoyed an acclaimed career working in many areas of dentistry, including clinical practice, teaching and research.

He co-authored a book titled <u>Mastering the Art of Complete Dentures</u>, and served as Assistant Professor of Prosthodontics at both the Harvard School of Dental Medicine in Boston, Massachusetts, and the University of Texas Health Science Center in San Antonio, Texas.

Following his early disability retirement from dentistry because of his life-threatening infections, Sandy held positions as a disability insurance specialist, co-owner of a community newspaper, president of a marketing, advertising and research firm, and City Commissioner in Weston, Florida. Toward the end of his professional career, Sandy was employed as a dental consultant for the Florida Department of Health in Tallahassee, Florida, where he worked in two key areas: public health dentistry and prosecution services, where he reviewed consumer patient complaints made against dentists.

Since receiving his Alzheimer's diagnosis in 2010, Sandy has channeled

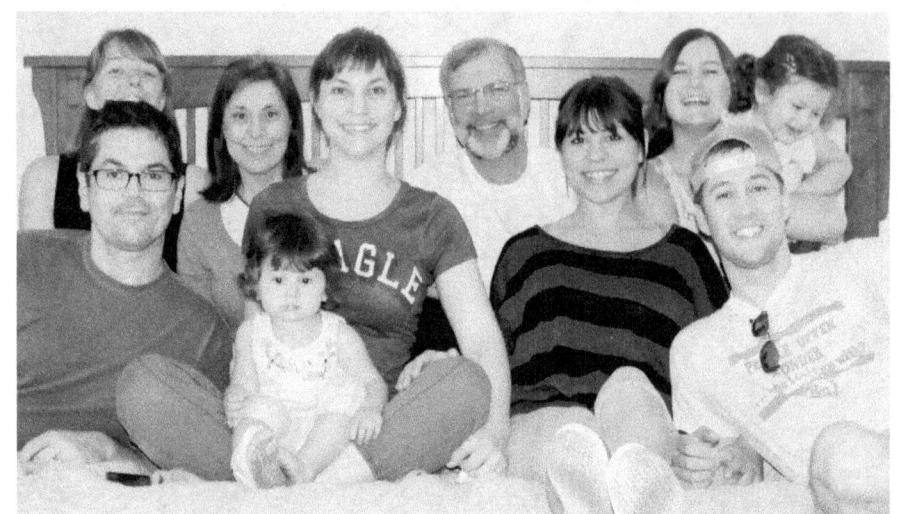

Our family, 2012

his energy and expertise into increasing awareness, raising funds for curative research, encouraging and advocating for patients and caregivers, and working to help decrease the stigma associated with this cognitive impairment.

While serving as an adviser and now an alumni of the National Alzheimer's Association 2012-2013 Early Stage Advisory Group, Sandy has traveled nationwide, speaking with everyone from members of Congress to a variety of organizations and groups.

In 2013, the Alexander "Sandy" Halperin Research Fund was initiated at Florida State University's College of Medicine Center for Brain Repair, and Sandy was also selected to be the focus of a CNN documentary filmed by senior health care producers under the direction of Dr. Sanjay Gupta.

Sandy lives in Tallahassee, Florida, with his wife. They have two daughters and three grandchildren.

Gina Davidson grew up in Sheboygan, Wisconsin, and moved to Florida in 1986, where she attended Florida State University and graduated magna cum laude in Secondary English Education.

She has been a writer for more than 20 years, worked for 13 years in journalism (writing, advertising and design), and has taught language arts at the elementary and high-school levels. She is currently working on a memoir about her relationship with her alcoholic, homeless, biological father whose fatal accident brought her life full circle.

She lives in Tallahassee, Florida, with her husband, their two children, and their golden retriever, Clark.

Current Symptoms Body Chart

Patient Name __Sandy Halperin__ Date __/__/__

My Right Side

Cervical spinal stenosis & disc problems

Daily neck & mid-thoracic pain, tingling,

numbness to arms & hands

Coronary artery calcifications/

plaques, confirmed by CT Scan

Thoracic Outlet Syndrome (?) with loss

of pulse on elbow and hand elevation

Barrett's Esophagus w/nausea & pain

Two prior surgeries:

Dec. 13, 2010 for synovial cyst,

disc herniations & Dec. 24, 2010

for CSF leak. Prior spinal fusion L45 S1 in 1968

Current post-surgery stenosis

Chronic and acute exacerbations/pain & sciat-

ica, numbness/tingling/burning to feet

Moderate pain in joints of hands, feet/toes,

generalized body osteoarthritis

Gall bladder removed March 3, 2012

Inguinal hernias, right and left R and L sides

Exacerbating, debilitating full-body fatigue

My Left Side

Cognitive impairments (Early Stage Alzheimer's)

Frequent, persistent, severe bronchial &/or sinus

infections requiring antibiotic therapy for many years

• Thickened & inflamed ethmoid, frontal &

maxillary sinuses, confirmed by MRI

Dramatic asthma, & hyperreactive airways,

Mayo Clinic "Methacholine Challenge Test"

• Thickened, inflamed bronchial walls,

Bronchiectasis, Atelectasisa in

lower left lung lobe,

all confirmed by CT Scan

Bilateral Ulnar Nerve

Compression and Brachial Plexus

involvements with intense pain

Carpal Tunnel Nerve Compression (R & L)

Button TURP prostate surgery, May 3, 2011

Overactive bladder, will need 2nd prostate surgery

• 8 mm+ kidney stone in L kidney,

confirmed by CT Scans/tomography radiographs

Secondary erythrocytosis & thrombocytopenia

as confirmed by bone biopsy, blood tests,

including iron and/or ferretin levels

& clinical symptoms

Lower GI symptoms of constipation & diarrhea

Notes

Notes